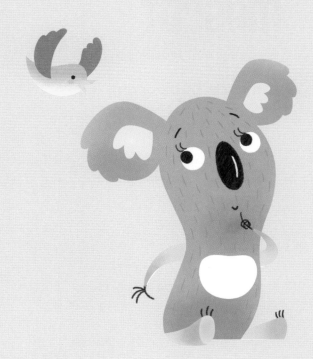

To our Kickstarter backers (thank you!)
and anyone with a little Chloe in them

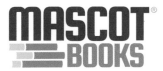

www.mascotbooks.com

Chloe Has Chlamydia

©2018 Jackie Prince. All Rights Reserved. No part of this publication may be reproduced, stored in a retrieval system or transmitted in any form by any means electronic, mechanical, or photocopying, recording or otherwise without the permission of the author.

For more information, please contact:
Mascot Books
620 Herndon Parkway #320
Herndon, VA 20170
info@mascotbooks.com

Library of Congress Control Number: 2018901858

CPSIA Code: PRTWP0318A
ISBN-13: 978-1-68401-832-1

Printed in Malaysia

Chloe Has
Chlamydia

by
Jackie Prince

illustrated by
Liesje Kraai

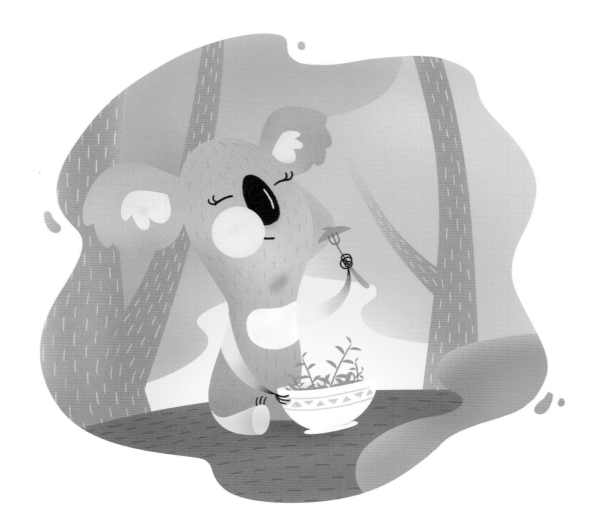

Chloe is a koala.

She lives in Gippsland, Australia, in a eucalyptus tree. YUM!

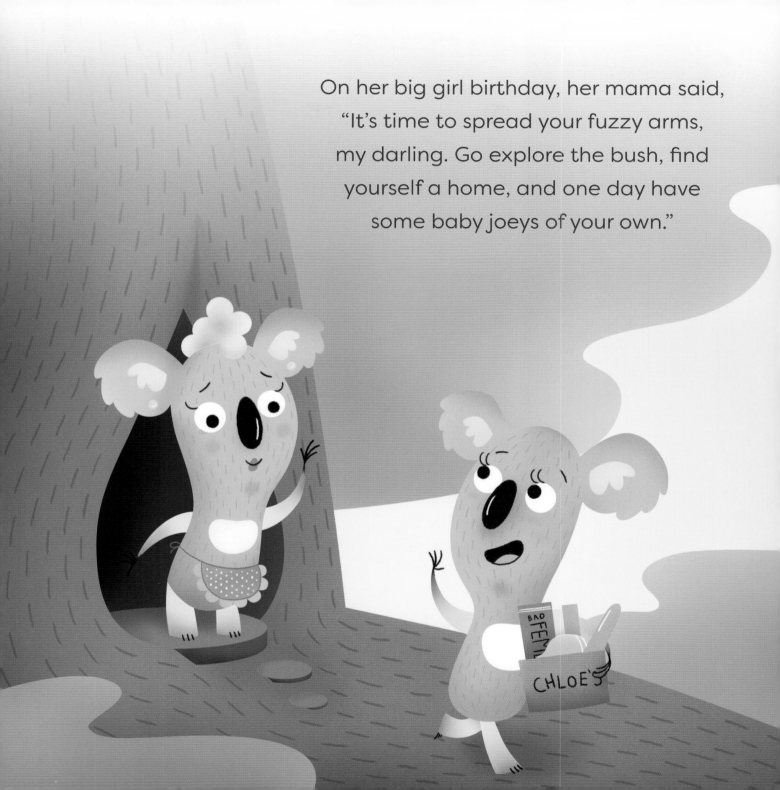

On her big girl birthday, her mama said, "It's time to spread your fuzzy arms, my darling. Go explore the bush, find yourself a home, and one day have some baby joeys of your own."

Hunting for roommates was a *biatch.*

#Fail

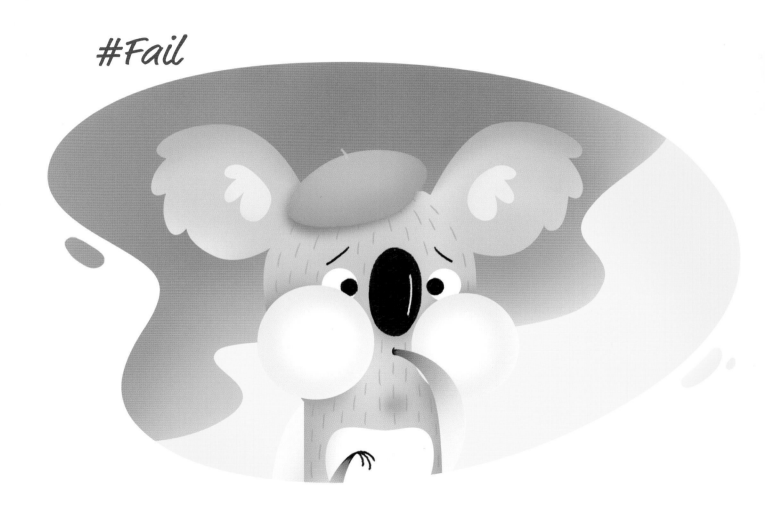

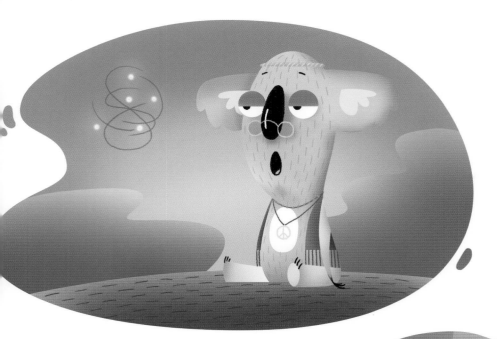

#DoubleFail

#WhatIsEven
HappeningHere

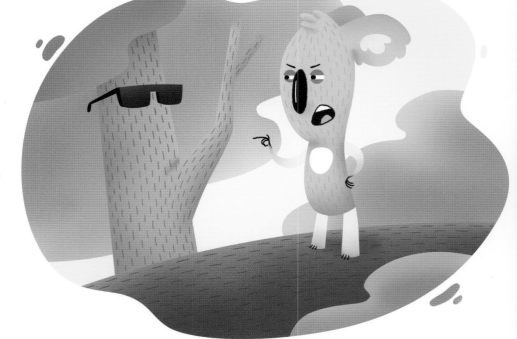

But after a few unsuccessful attempts . . .

Chloe found the perfect spot in a lush eucalyptus tree all her own and went to sleep.

Aaaahhhhh.

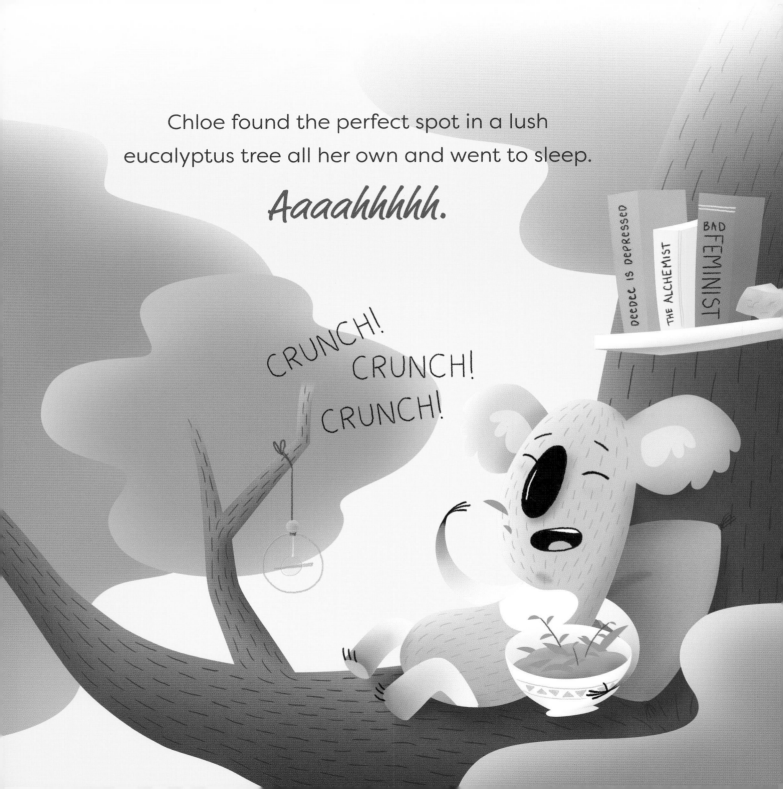

One steamy summer evening, Chloe heard loud,
deep bellows coming from her left and her right.

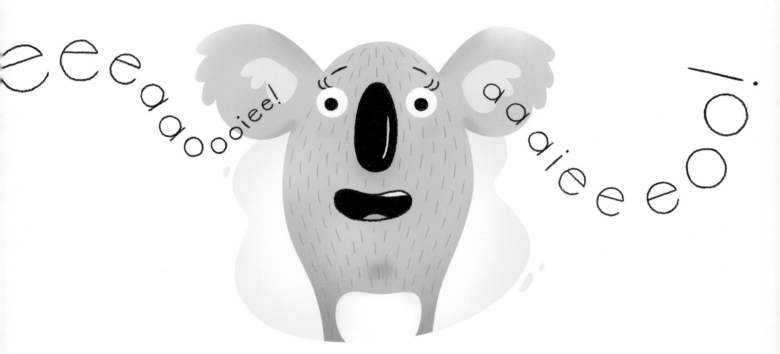

Oh boy! she thought. *Mating season!*

The sounds led Chloe to a hot piece named Tim.

"How ya goin'?" she asked.

"Alright!" replied Tim. "I like leaves!"

"Me too!" Chloe said, her nature's pocket tingling.

"Let's mate, mate!"

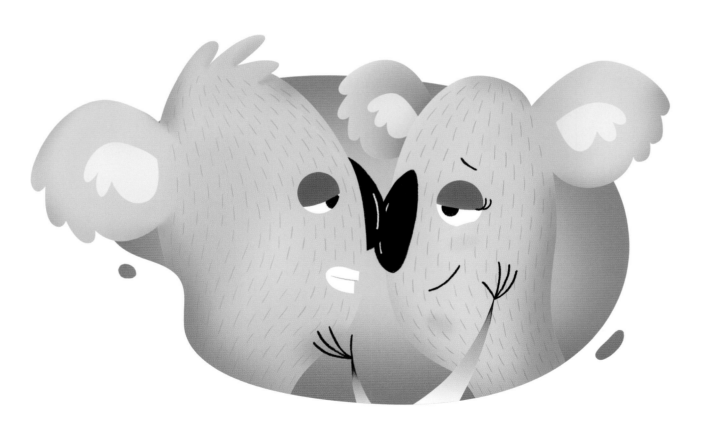

"That was fun!"

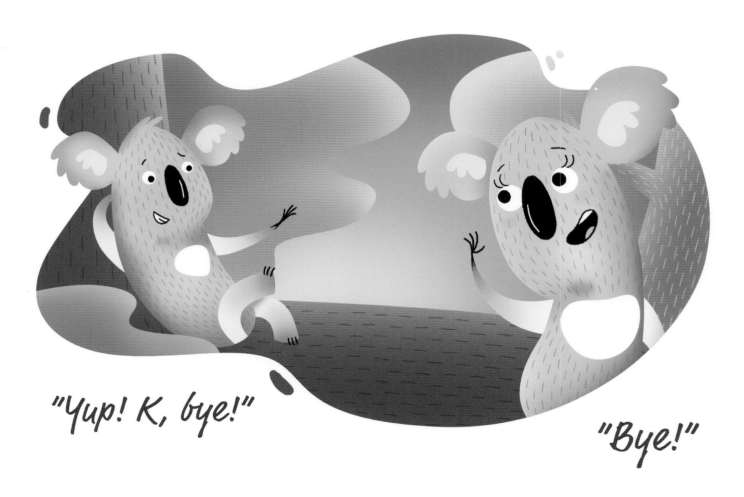

"Yup! K, bye!"

"Bye!"

Chloe climbed back into her tree
and fell asleep, satisfied with herself
and excited to meet her baby joey
in just a few months.

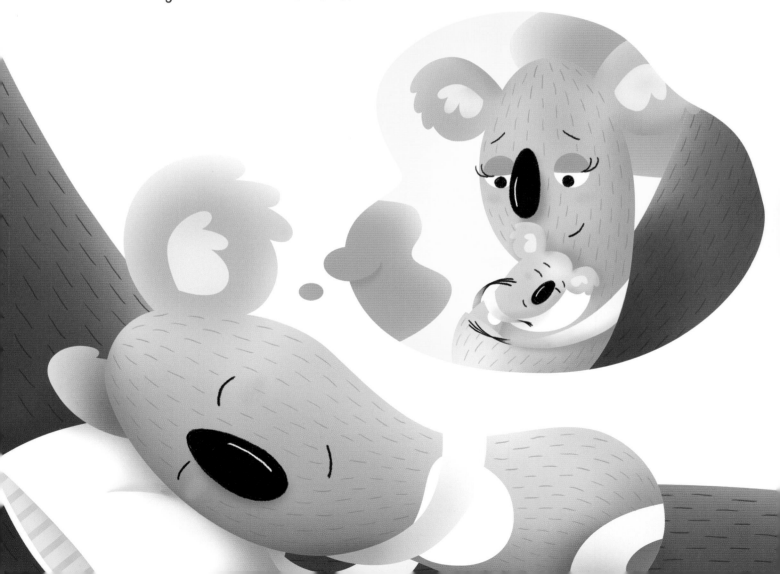

Some weeks later, Chloe was napping, having a saucy dream about a koala who had been sexting her. She felt a tingle and woke up to pee. It burned like the time she front slid down a rough branch.

"Hmm," Chloe muttered, "maybe I ate some bad eucalyptus leaves . . ."

She spent the next few days eating from the other side of her tree, but it still felt like she was peeing Sriracha sauce. *Strange.*

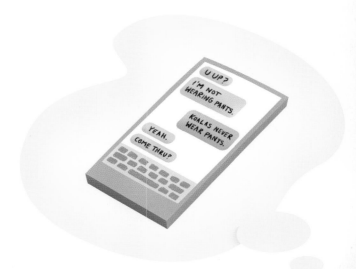

Chloe climbed over to Dr. Honeyeater's office, who took some tests.

"Oh boy." She let out a sigh. "Chloe, it appears you've got chlamydia."

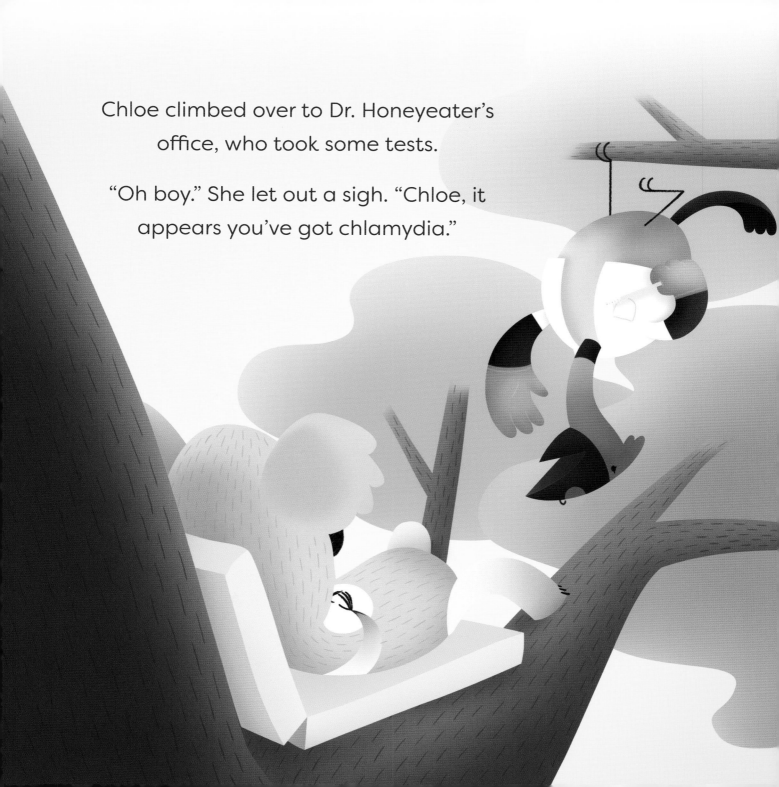

"Uh . . . *what's chlamydia?"*

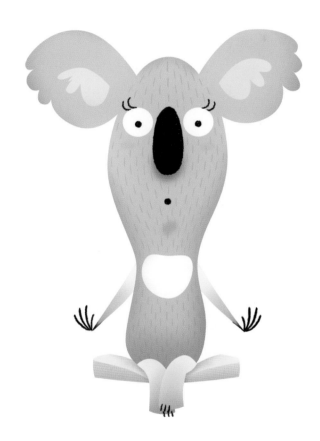

"It's a common sexually transmitted infection, or STI, that's passed along during unprotected vaginal, anal, or oral sex."

"All the sexes!" Chloe exclaimed.

"Chloe," Dr. Honeyeater asked, "have you been playing hide the snake with other koalas?"

"Never!" Chloe replied. "Snakes are poisonous!"

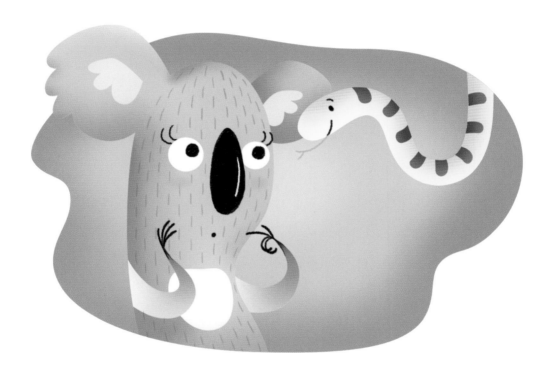

"You know," Dr. Honeyeater continued, "pounding the pouch, wetting the woodlands, burying the wombat, sharpening the scissors?"

"Ohhh, bumping fuzzies! I have, Dr. Honeyeater . . ."

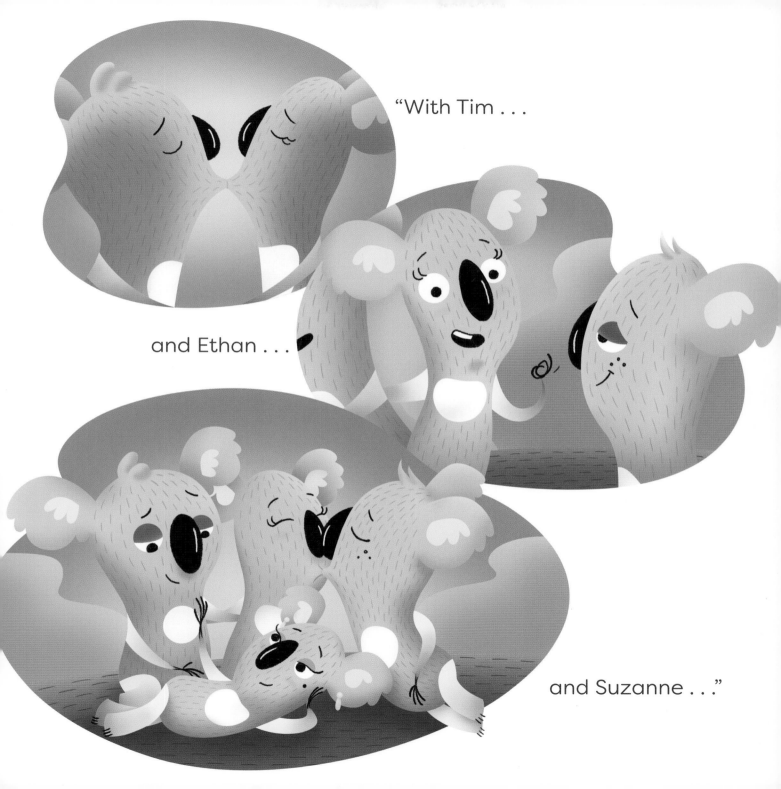

"With Tim . . .

and Ethan . . .

and Suzanne . . ."

"I see," Dr. Honeyeater replied. "Lucky for you, we might be able to treat it since we caught it early. But, chlamydia can damage your reproductive system, so there is a chance you won't be able to have baby joeys."

Chloe was distraught. After all, a big part of growing up is having a family of your own. Or so she thought.

What would Mama think? What about the other gossipy koalas with their growing joey bumps?

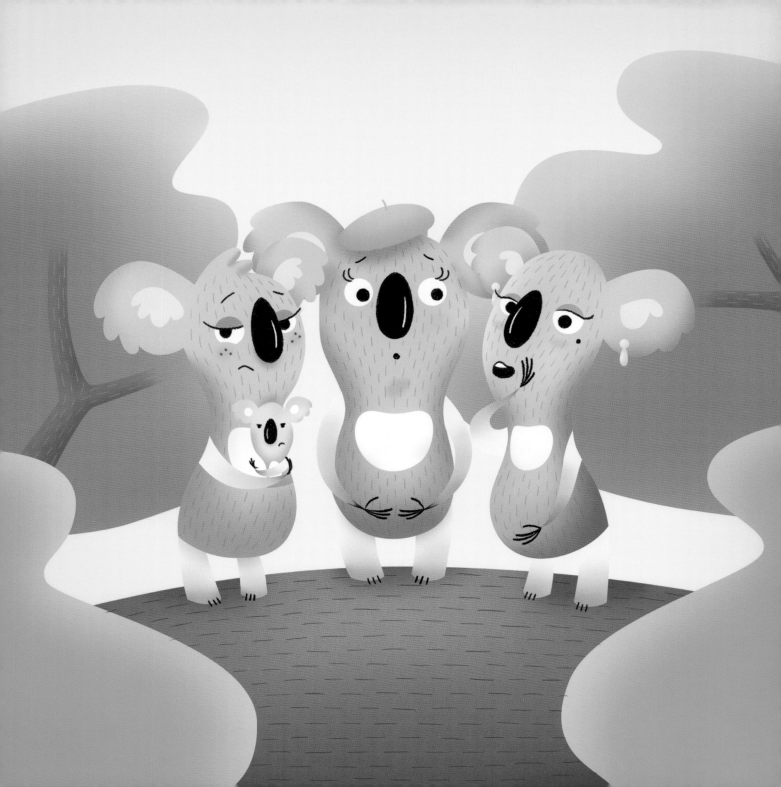

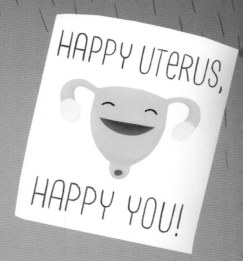

HAPPY UTERUS, HAPPY YOU!

"But Dr. Honeyeater," Chloe wailed, "none of my sex friends told me they have chlamydia!"

"Well, Chloe, it's possible they don't know. Most koalas have no symptoms. Even if they do, they can take weeks to appear. Like a stinging sensation when you pee, pelvic pain during sex, or everyone's favorite . . .

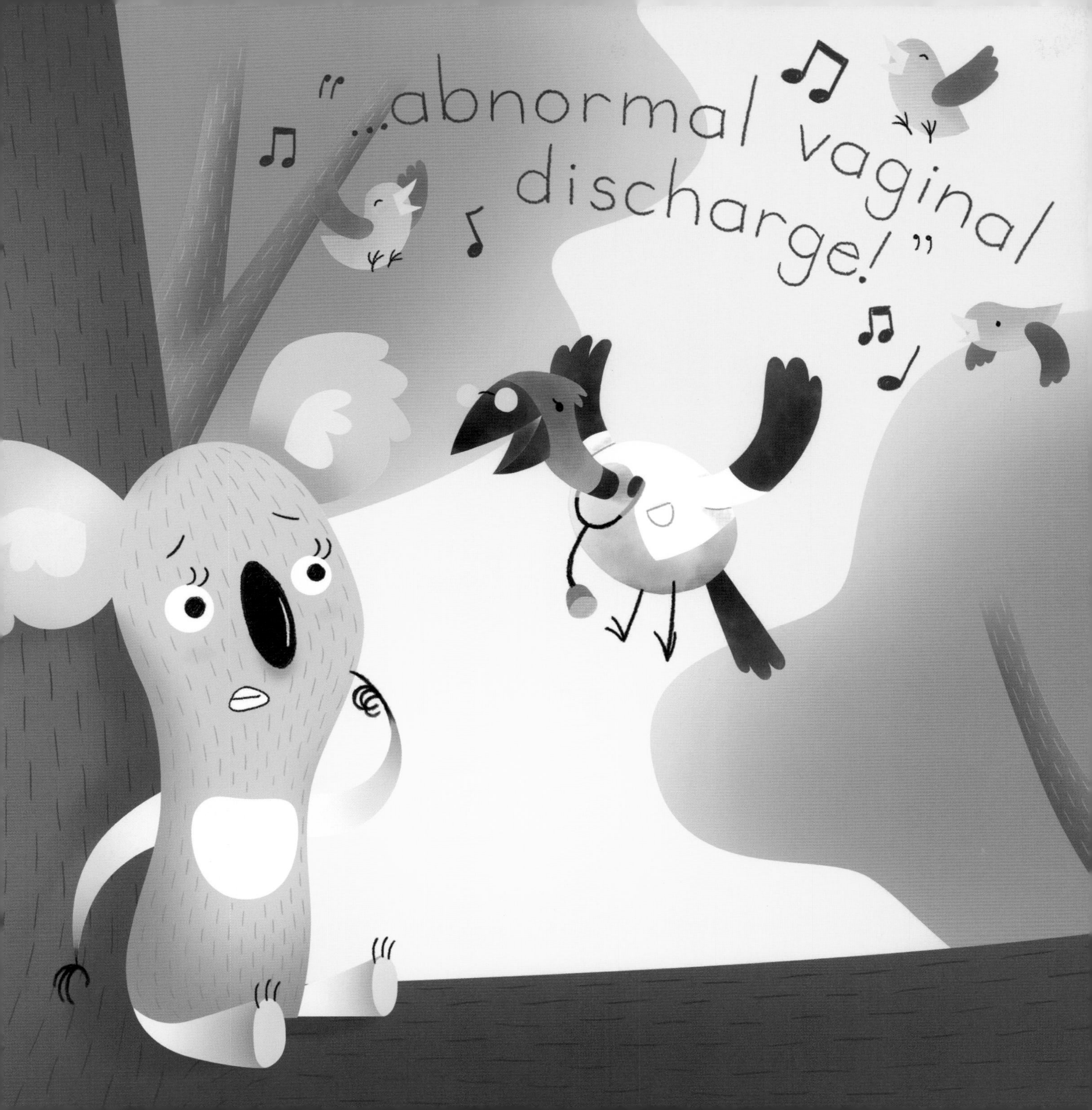
"...abnormal vaginal discharge!"

"Better give your sexy mates the news, Chloe, and tell them to get screened and practice safe sex. But no sex for you until you've kicked *the* C to the curb. Come back and see me when you've finished these antibiotics. And for non-baby-making sex, always use . . ."

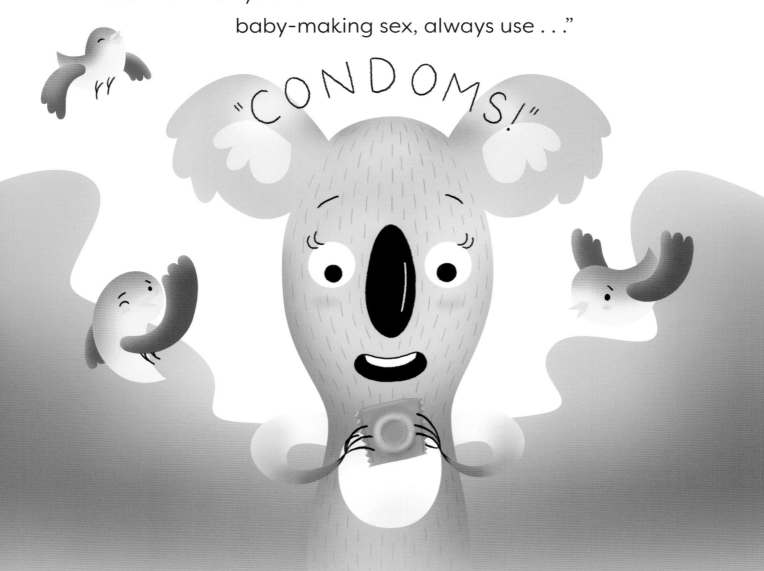

"CONDOMS!"

Chloe found Tim at Possum's Pub and broke the news to him.

"Oy, I had no idea. Very sorry, Chloe. I hope you can still have joeys, mate!"

"Me too," said Chloe. "K, bye."

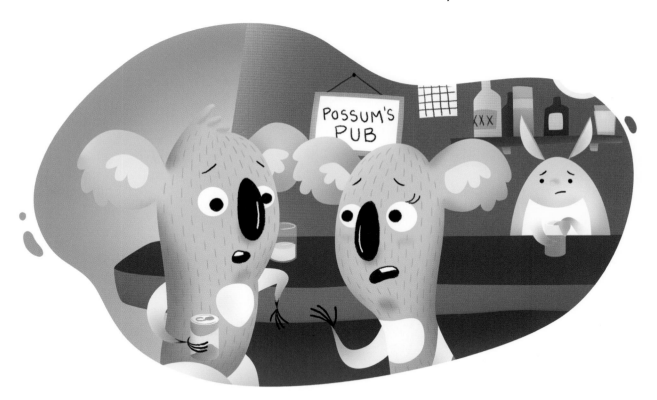

Chloe stopped by Ethan's tree, too, and paid Suzanne an *extra*-long visit. They thanked her for letting them know and promised to make appointments to see Dr. Honeyeater to get screened.

That evening, Chloe stress-ate a few too many leaves, anxious about her chlamydia.

She thought back to something Dr. Honeyeater had said:
"Most koalas have no symptoms."

Suddenly, Chloe thought about all her friends who might not know they have chlamydia and were mating without protection, passing STIs around like an old, beat-up rugby ball.

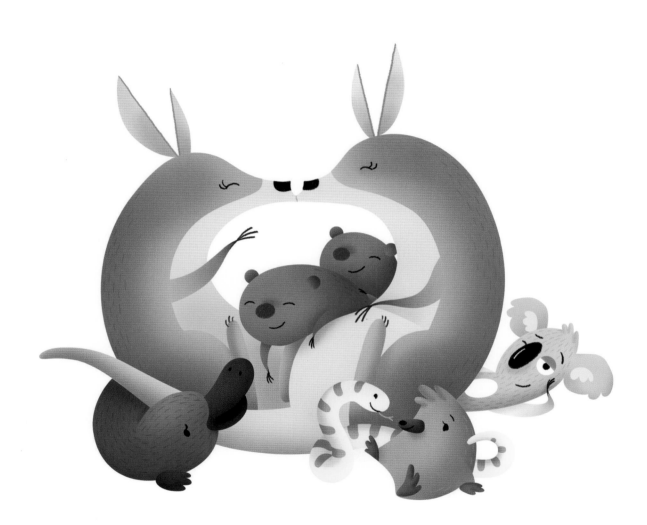

The next morning, Chloe woke up with a mission. She shoved a bunch of condoms into her pouch and made her way into the forest.

She approached a koala caressing a cockatoo.

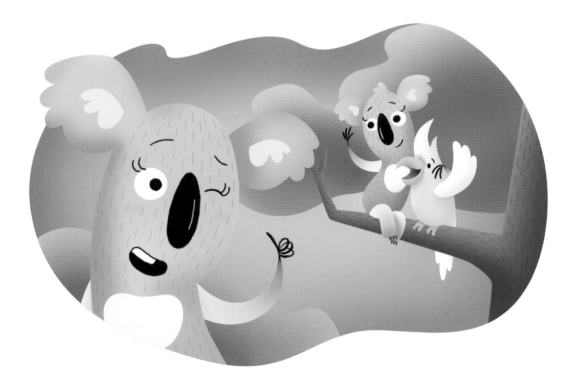

"Hi! I'm Chloe, and I have chlamydia, and maybe you do too. Glad I caught you just in time. *Here are some condoms!*"

"Thanks, mate!" they called after her.

Chloe arrived at the next tree where three koalas were touching each other and listening to "Sexual Healing."

"Hi! I'm Chloe, and I have chlamydia, and maybe you do too. Glad I caught you just in time. *Here are some condoms!*"

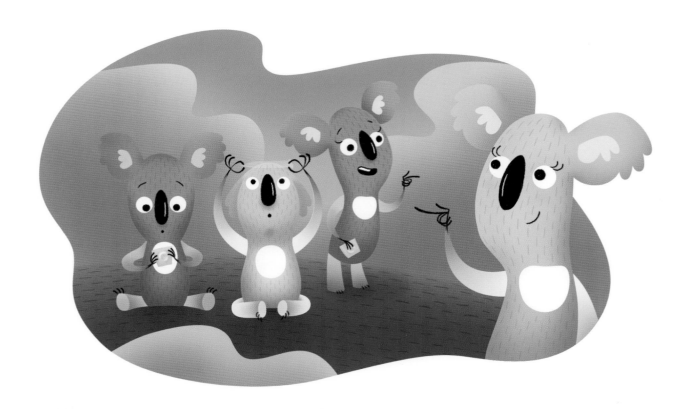

"Thanks, mate!" they called after her.

The next tree was beautiful and filled with tons of delicious-looking leaves, some painted red with berries.

"Hayyy," a beautiful koala greeted Chloe. "I'm Darlene."

"Hey!" replied Chloe. "Your tree is dazzling. I'm Chloe, and—"

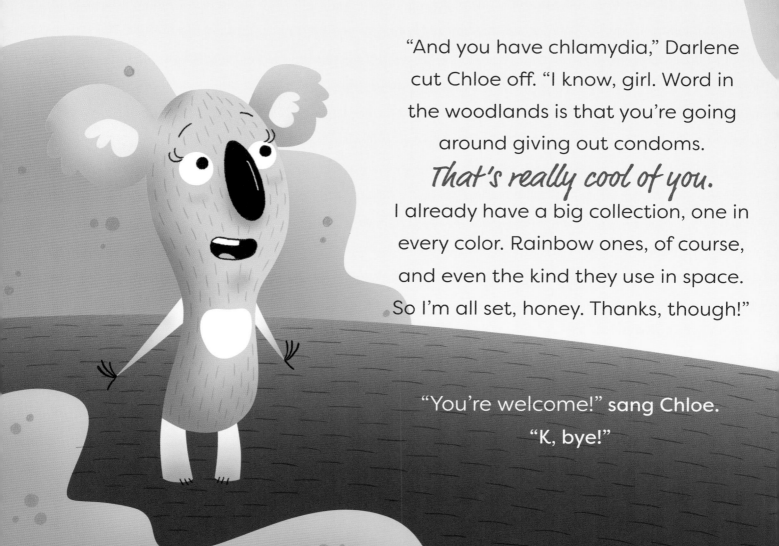

"And you have chlamydia," Darlene cut Chloe off. "I know, girl. Word in the woodlands is that you're going around giving out condoms. *That's really cool of you.* I already have a big collection, one in every color. Rainbow ones, of course, and even the kind they use in space. So I'm all set, honey. Thanks, though!"

"You're welcome!" sang Chloe.
"K, bye!"

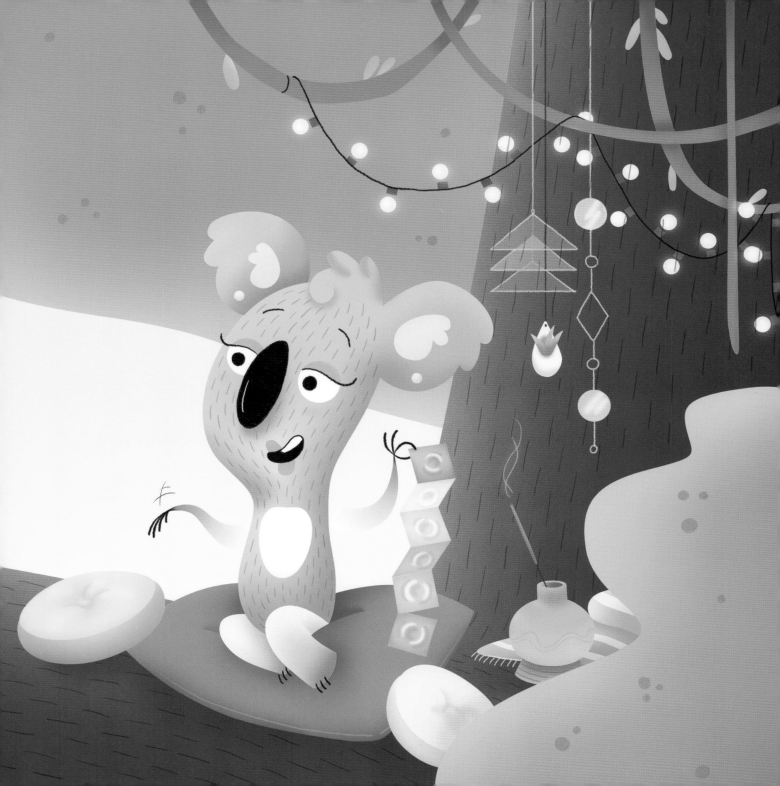

Chloe got home that evening tired but happy. She had taught a bunch of koalas about chlamydia and handed out enough condoms to cover a dolphin dick— and those things are huge.

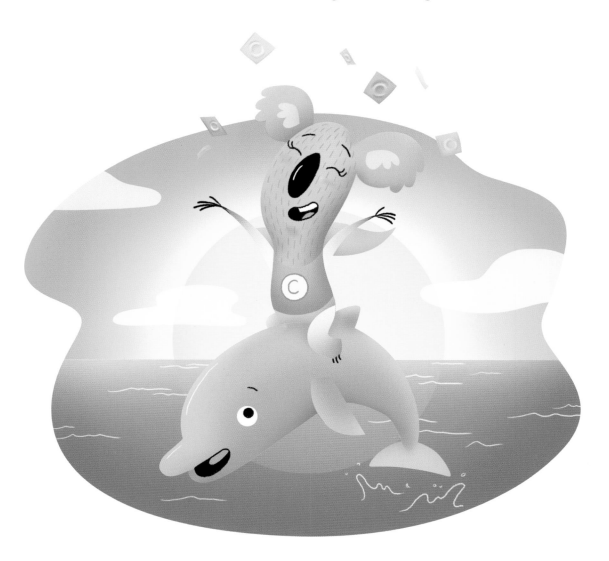

The next day, Chloe went for her follow-up visit with Dr. Honeyeater. She was nervous but hopeful.

Dr. Honeyeater checked Chloe out and broke into song.

"Great news, Chloe!" she exclaimed.

"It looks like you've kicked your chlamydia!"

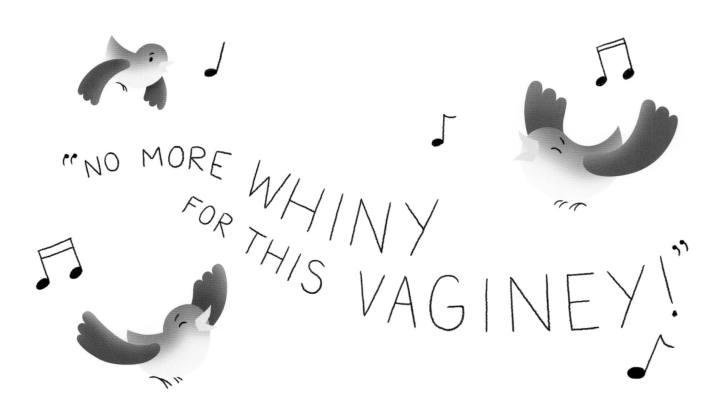

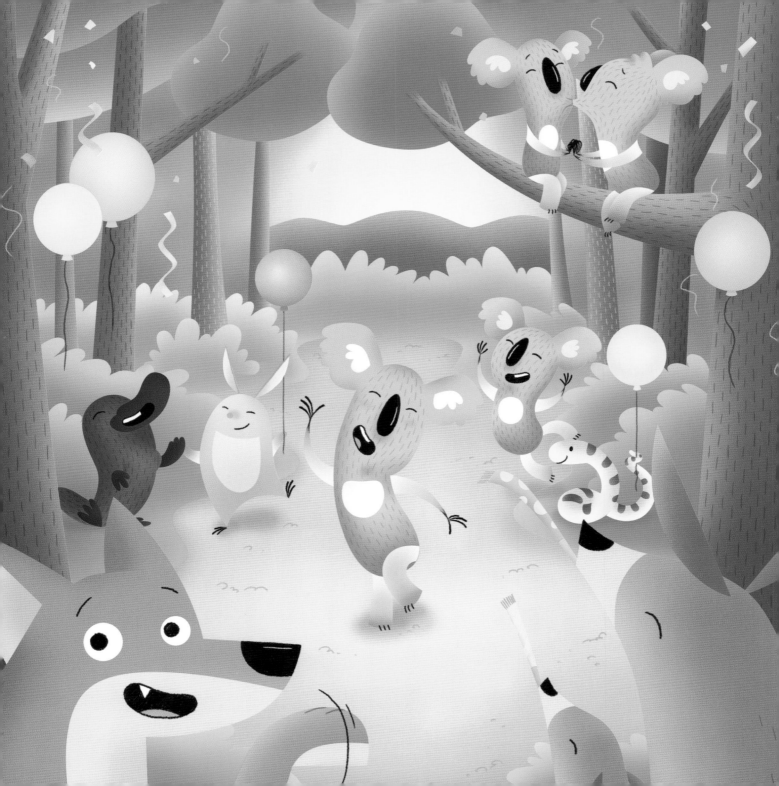

"*YASSSS!*" cried Chloe, feeling ecstatic. She imagined a dance sequence around her, with all of her outback friends cheering and holding balloons.

"So," asked Dr. Honeyeater, "are you going to try and have some little joeys now?"

"Maybe someday, Doc. First I want to keep spreading the word about chlamydia so all my mates can mate safely without passing or catching *the C.*"

"Wonderful, Chloe! And make sure you keep coming back for check-ups!"

Chloe smiled as the sun set over Gippsland. It was good to be home. She settled into her favorite branch and prepared for an epic nap.

"Hi," she said to no one in particular. "I'm Chloe, and I don't have chlamydia."

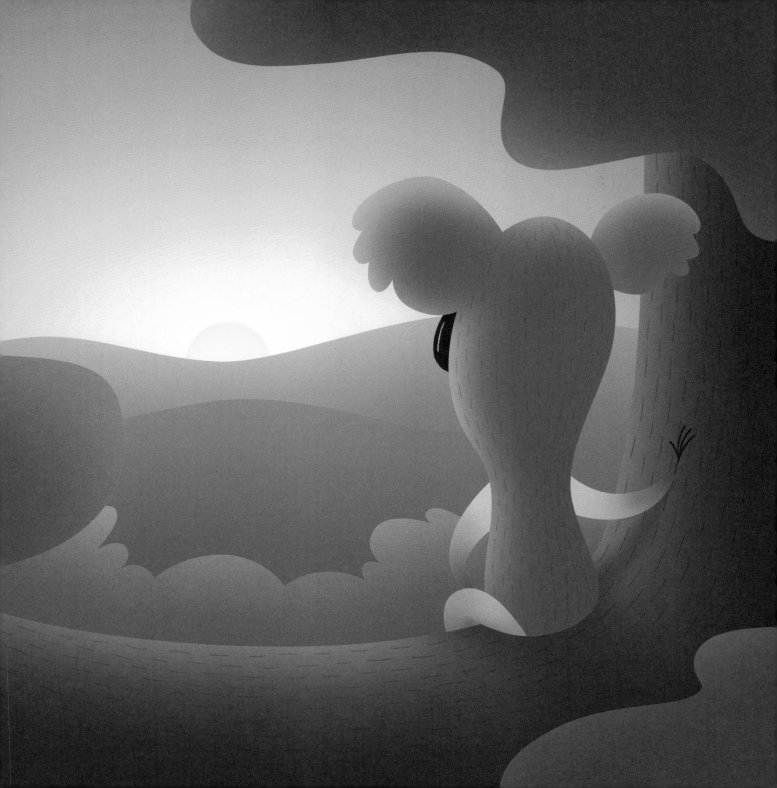

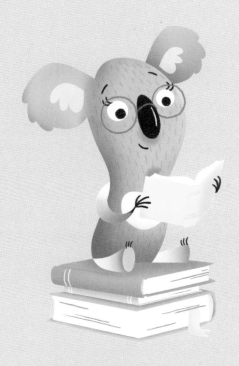

Hi, I'm Chloe,

and I don't have chlamydia anymore! But I used to!
And you could get it, too, if you don't protect your bod.
So spread the word—not STIs.